The Keto Vegetarian Healthy Lifestyle

Live Longer and Be Fit with Balanced Tasty Recipes

Lauren Bellisario

Table of Contents

Soy Chorizo, Eggs & Feta Cheese Plate

Preparation time: 10 minutes

Cooking time: 5 minutes

Serving: 4

Nutritional Values (Per Serving):

- Calories:414
- Total Fat: 34.7g
- Saturated Fat:19.3 g
- Total Carbs: 2 g
- Dietary Fiber:0 g
- Sugar: 0g
- Protein: 24g
- Sodium: 639mg

Ingredients:

- 1 tsp olive oil
- 1 tsp smoked paprika

- 3 oz soy chorizo, diced
- 4 eggs
- ½ cup crumbled feta cheese
- 2 green onions, thinly sliced diagonally
- 2 tbsp fresh parsley, chopped
- Greek yogurt to serve

Directions:

1. Preheat the oven to 350 F.
2. On a stovetop over medium temperature, heat the olive oil along with the paprika in an oven safe non- stick frying pan for 30 seconds. Add the soy chorizo and cook until lightly browned; spoon the soy chorizo into a bowl, leaving the olive oil in the pan.
3. Crack the eggs into the pan, cook for 2 minutes, and then sprinkle with the chorizo and crumble the feta cheese all around the egg white, but not on the yolks.
4. Transfer the pan to the oven and bake for 1 to 2 more minutes or until the yolks are quite set, but still runny within.
5. Remove the pan, garnish with the green onions and parsley.
6. Serve warm with Greek yogurt.

Croque Madame with Pesto

Preparation time: 15 minutes

Cooking time: 30 minutes

Serving: 4

Nutritional Values (Per Serving):

- Calories: 208
- Total Fat: 15.3g
- Saturated Fat:3 g
- Total Carbs: 12 g
- Dietary Fiber: 5g
- Sugar: 3g
- Protein: 8g
- Sodium: 73mg

Ingredients:
For the béchamel:

- 2 tbsp unsalted butter
- 1 cup almond milk + extra as needed
- 2 tbsp almond flour
- Salt and black pepper to season
- ½ tsp nutmeg powder

- 4 tbsp grated cheddar cheese

For the pesto:

- ½ cup basil leaves
- 1/3 cup toasted pine nuts
- ¼ cup grated parmesan cheese
- 1 garlic clove, peeled
- ¼ cup olive oil

For the sandwich:

- 2 tbsp melted butter
- 4 slices low carb bread
- 1 (7 oz) can sliced mushrooms, drained
- 3 medium tomatoes, sliced
- 4 slices mozzarella cheese
- 1 tbsp olive oil
- 4 large whole eggs
- Baby arugula for garnishing

Directions:

For the béchamel sauce:

1. Heat the butter and half of the milk in a medium saucepan over medium heat. When the butter melts, whisk in the remaining milk with flour until smooth roux forms.

2. Season with salt, black pepper, and nutmeg. Reduce the heat to low and stir in the cheddar cheese until melted. Turn the heat off and set the sauce aside.

For the pesto:

3. In a food processor, puree the basil, pine nuts, parmesan, garlic, and olive oil.

4. Transfer to a glass jar, cover the lid, and refrigerate until ready to use. For the sandwich:

5. Preheat the grill to medium-high.

6. Brush both sides of each bread with butter and toast each on both sides until golden.

7. Remove onto a plate and spread the béchamel sauce on one side of each bread, then the pesto, and divide the mushrooms, tomatoes, and mozzarella cheese on top of each bread.

8. One after the other, return each sandwich to the grill and cook until the cheese melts. Transfer to serving plates.

9. Heat the olive oil in a skillet over medium heat and crack an egg into the oil. Cook until the whites are set but the yolks still soft and runny. Place the egg on a sandwich and repeat the same process for the remaining eggs for the rest of the sandwich.

10. Season with salt and black pepper, and garnish with the arugula.

11. Serve warm.

Seitan Tex-Mex Casserole

Preparation time: 5 minutes

Cooking time: 35 minutes

Serving: 4

Nutritional Values (Per Serving):

- Calories: 464
- Total Fat:37.8 g
- Saturated Fat:7.4 g
- Total Carbs: 12 g
- Dietary Fiber: 2g
- Sugar: 3g, Protein:24 g
- Sodium: 147mg

Ingredients:

- 2 tbsp butter

- 1 ½ lb seitan
- 3 tbsp Tex-Mex seasoning
- 2 tbsp chopped jalapeño peppers
- ½ cup crushed tomatoes
- Salt and black pepper to taste
- ½ cup shredded provolone cheese
- 1 tbsp chopped fresh green onion to garnish
- 1 cup sour cream for serving

Directions:

1. Preheat the oven and grease a baking dish with cooking spray. Set aside.
2. Melt the butter in a medium skillet over medium heat and cook the seitan until brown, 10 minutes.
3. Stir in the Tex-Mex seasoning, jalapeño peppers, and tomatoes; simmer for 5 minutes and adjust the taste with salt and black pepper.
4. Transfer and level the mixture in the baking dish. Top with the provolone cheese and bake in the upper rack of the oven for 15 to 20 minutes or until the cheese melts and is golden brown.
5. Remove the dish and garnish with the green onion.
6. Serve the casserole with sour cream.

Tofu Loco Moco

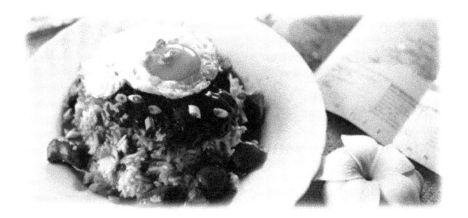

Preparation time: 12 minutes

Cooking time: 28 minutes

Serving: 4

Nutritional Values (Per Serving):

- Calories: 258
- Total Fat: 21g
- Saturated Fat: 13.5g
- Total Carbs: 16 g
- Dietary Fiber: 6g

- Sugar: 7g
- Protein: 6g
- Sodium:37 mg

Ingredients:

For the loco moco patties:

- 1 ½ lb tofu, crumbled
- 1/3 cup almond meal
- ½ tsp nutmeg powder
- 1 tsp onion powder
- Salt and black pepper to taste
- 1 large egg
- 2 tbsp cashew cream
- 3 tbsp avocado oil

For the mushroom gravy:

- 1 tbsp salted butter
- 1 shallot, finely chopped
- 1 cup sliced oyster mushrooms
- 1 cup vegetable stock
- 2 tsp tamarind sauce
- Salt and black pepper to taste

- ½ tsp arrowroot starch

For the fried eggs:

- 2 tbsp olive oil
- 4 large eggs
- Salt and black pepper to taste

Directions:

For the loco moco patties:

1. In a large bowl, combine the tofu, almond meal, nutmeg powder, onion powder, salt, and black pepper. In a small bowl, whisk the eggs with the cashew cream and mix into the tofu mixture until the batter is sticky. Form 8 patties from the mixture.
2. Heat the avocado oil in a medium skillet over medium heat and fry the patties in batches on both sides until compacted and cooked through, 16 minutes. Transfer to a serving plate and set aside.

For the mushroom gravy:

1. Melt the butter in the same skillet and cook the shallot and mushrooms until softened, 7 minutes.

2. Meanwhile, in a medium bowl, combine the remaining Ingredients and pour the mixture into the skillet. Cook until slightly thickened, 3 minutes.
3. Turn the heat off and set aside. For the fried eggs:
4. Heat half of the olive oil in a small skillet, crack in an egg, and fry sunshine style, 1 minute. Plate and fry the remaining eggs in the same manner. Season with salt and black pepper.
5. Serve the tofu with the mushroom gravy and the fried rice.

Baked Mushrooms with Creamy Brussels Sprouts

Preparation time: 8 minutes

Cooking time: 2 hours 35 minutes

Serving: 4

Nutritional Values (Per Serving):

- Calories: 492
- Total Fat: 37.9g
- Saturated Fat: 9.1g
- Total Carbs: 13g
- Dietary Fiber:2 g
- Sugar:2 g
- Protein: 29g
- Sodium: 779mg

Ingredients:

For the mushrooms:

- 1 lb whole white button mushrooms
- Salt and black pepper to taste
- 2 tsp dried thyme
- 1 bay leaf
- 5 black peppercorns
- ½ cups vegetable broth
- 2 garlic cloves, minced
- 1 ½ oz fresh ginger, grated
- 1 tbsp coconut oil
- 1 tbsp smoked paprika

For the creamy Brussel sprouts:

- ½ lb Brussel sprouts, halved
- 1 ½ cups cashew cream
- Salt and ground black pepper to taste

Directions:

For the mushroom roast:

1. Preheat the oven to 200 F.

2. Pour all the mushroom Ingredients into a baking dish, stir well, and cover with foil. Bake in the oven until softened, 1 to 2 hours.

3. Remove the dish, take off the foil, and use a slotted spoon to fetch the mushrooms onto serving plates. Set aside.

For the creamy Brussel sprouts:

1. Pour the broth in the baking dish into a medium pot and add the Brussel sprouts. Add about ½ cup of water if needed and cook for 7 to 10 minutes or until softened.

2. Stir in the cashew cream, adjust the taste with salt and black pepper, and simmer for 15 minutes.

3. Serve the creamy Brussel sprouts with the mushrooms.

Pimiento Tofu balls

Preparation time: 10 minutes

Cooking time: 15 minutes

Serving: 4

Nutritional Values (Per Serving):

- Calories:254
- Total Fat: 36.8g
- Saturated Fat: 8.7g
- Total Carbs: 12g
- Dietary Fiber: 1g
- Sugar: 1g
- Protein:26 g
- Sodium:773 mg

Ingredients:

- ¼ cup chopped pimientos
- 1/3 cup mayonnaise
- 3 tbsp cashew cream

- 1 tsp paprika powder
- 1 pinch cayenne pepper
- 1 tbsp Dijon mustard
- 4 oz grated Parmesan cheese
- 1 ½ lbs. tofu, pressed and crumbled
- Salt and black pepper to taste
- 1 large egg
- 2 tbsp olive oil, for frying

Directions:

1. In a large bowl, add all the Ingredients except for the olive oil and with gloves on your hands, mix the Ingredients until well combined. Form bite size balls from the mixture.
2. Heat the olive oil in a medium non-stick skillet and fry the tofu balls in batches on both sides until brown and cooked through, 4 to 5 minutes on each side.
3. Transfer the tofu balls to a serving plate and serve warm.

Tempeh with Garlic Asparagus

Preparation time: 10 minutes

Cooking time: 18 minutes

Serving: 4

Nutritional Values (Per Serving):

- Calories: 181
- Total Fat:17.5 g
- Saturated Fat:11 g
- Total Carbs: 6 g
- Dietary Fiber: 3g
- Sugar: 2g
- Protein: 3g
- Sodium: 140mg

Ingredients:

For the tempeh:

- 3 tbsp butter
- 4 tempeh slices
- Salt and black pepper to taste

For the garlic buttered asparagus:

- 2 tbsp. olive oil
- 2 garlic cloves, minced
- 1 lb asparagus, trimmed and halved
- Salt and black pepper to taste
- 1 tbsp dried parsley
- 1 small lemon, juiced

Directions:

For the tempeh:

1. Melt the butter in a medium skillet over medium heat, season the tempeh with salt, black pepper and fry in the butter on both sides until brown and cooked through, 10 minutes. Transfer to a plate and set aside in a warmer for serving.

For the garlic asparagus:

1. Heat the olive oil in a medium skillet over medium heat, and sauté the garlic until fragrant, 30 seconds.
2. Stir in the asparagus, season with salt and black pepper, and cook until slightly softened with a bit of crunch, 5 minutes.

3. Mix in the parsley, lemon juice, toss to coat well, and plate the asparagus.

4. Serve the asparagus warm with the tempeh.

Mushroom Curry Pie

Preparation time: 15 minutes

Cooking time: 55 minutes

Serving: 4

Nutritional Values (Per Serving):

- Calories:548
- Total Fat: 55.9g
- Saturated Fat:8.5 g
- Total Carbs: 6g
- Dietary Fiber:2 g
- Sugar: 2g
- Protein:8 g
- Sodium: 405mg

Ingredients:

For the piecrust:

- 1 tbsp flax seed powder + 3 tbsp water
- ¾ cup coconut flour
- 4 tbsp chia seeds

- 4 tbsp almond flour
- 1 tbsp psyllium husk powder
- 1 tsp baking powder
- 1 pinch salt
- 3 tbsp olive oil
- 4 tbsp water

For the filling:

- 1 cup chopped cremini mushrooms
- 1 cup vegan mayonnaise
- 3 tbsp + 9 tbsp water
- ½ red bell pepper, finely chopped
- 1 tsp turmeric powder
- ½ tsp paprika powder
- ½ tsp garlic powder
- ¼ tsp black pepper
- ½ cup cashew cream
- 1¼ cups shredded tofu cheese

Directions:

1. In two separate bowls, mix the different portions of flax seed powder with the respective quantity of water and set aside to absorb for 5 minutes.

2. Preheat the oven to 350 F.

3. Make the crust:

4. When the flax egg is ready, pour the smaller quantity into a food processor, add the coconut flour, chia seeds, almond flour, psyllium husk powder, baking powder, salt, olive oil, and water. Blend the Ingredients until a ball forms out of the dough.

5. Line a springform pan with an 8-inch diameter parchment paper and grease the pan with cooking spray.

6. Spread the dough in the bottom of the pan and bake in the oven for 15 minutes.

Make the filling:

1. In a bowl, add the remaining flax egg, mushrooms, mayonnaise, water, bell pepper, turmeric, paprika, garlic powder, black pepper, cashew cream, and tofu cheese. Combine the mixture evenly and fill the piecrust. Bake further for 40 minutes or until the pie is golden brown.

2. Remove, slice, and serve the pie with a chilled strawberry drink.

Spicy Cheese with Tofu Balls

Preparation time: 20 minutes

Cooking time: 20 minutes

Serving: 4

Nutritional Values (Per Serving):

- Calories: 259
- Total Fat: 55.9g
- Saturated Fat:11.4 g
- Total Carbs: 5 g
- Dietary Fiber: 1g
- Sugar: 1g
- Protein: 16g
- Sodium: 452mg

Ingredients:

For the spicy cheese:

- 1/3 cup vegan mayonnaise

- ¼ cup pickled jalapenos
- 1 tsp paprika powder
- 1 tbsp mustard powder
- 1 pinch cayenne pepper
- 4 oz grated tofu cheese

For the tofu balls:

- 1 tbsp flax seed powder + 3 tbsp water
- 2 ½ cup crumbled tofu
- Salt and black pepper
- 2 tbsp plant butter, for frying

Directions:

1. Make the spicy cheese. In a bowl, mix the mayonnaise, jalapenos, paprika, mustard powder, cayenne powder, and cheddar cheese. Set aside.
2. In another medium bowl, combine the flax seed powder with water and allow absorbing for 5 minutes.
3. Add the flax egg to the cheese mixture, the crumbled tofu, salt, and black pepper, and combine well. Use your hands to form large meatballs out of the mix.

4. Then, melt the butter in a large skillet over medium heat and fry the tofu balls until cooked and browned on the outside.

5. Serve the tofu balls with roasted cauliflower mash and mayonnaise.

Avocado Coconut Pie

Preparation time: 30 minutes

Cooking time: 50 minutes

Serving: 4

Nutritional Values (Per Serving):

- Calories:680
- Total Fat:71.8 g
- Saturated Fat:20.9 g
- Total Carbs: 10g
- Dietary Fiber:7 g
- Sugar: 2g
- Protein: 3g
- Sodium:525 mg

Ingredients:

For the piecrust:

- 1 tbsp flax seed powder + 3 tbsp water

- 4 tbsp coconut flour
- 4 tbsp chia seeds
- ¾ cup almond flour
- 1 tbsp psyllium husk powder
- 1 tsp baking powder
- 1 pinch salt
- 3 tbsp coconut oil
- 4 tbsp water

For the filling:

- 2 ripe avocados
- 1 cup vegan mayonnaise
- 3 tbsp flax seed powder + 9 tbsp water
- 2 tbsp fresh parsley, finely chopped
- 1 jalapeno, finely chopped
- ½ tsp onion powder
- ¼ tsp salt
- ½ cup cashew cream
- 1¼ cups shredded tofu cheese

Directions:

1. In 2 separate bowls, mix the different portions of flax seed powder with the respective quantity of water. Allow absorbing for 5 minutes.

2. Preheat the oven to 350 F.

3. In a food processor, add the coconut flour, chia seeds, almond flour, psyllium husk powder, baking powder, salt, coconut oil, water, and the smaller portion of the flax egg. Blend the Ingredients until the resulting dough forms into a ball.

4. Line a spring form pan with about 12-inch diameter of parchment paper and spread the dough in the pan. Bake for 10 to 15 minutes or until a light golden brown color is achieved.

5. Meanwhile, cut the avocado into halves lengthwise, remove the pit, and chop the pulp. Put in a bowl and add the mayonnaise, remaining flax egg, parsley, jalapeno, onion powder, salt, cashew cream, and tofu cheese. Combine well.

6. Remove the piecrust when ready and fill with the creamy mixture. Level the filling with a spatula and continue baking for 35 minutes or until lightly golden brown.

7. When ready, take out. Cool before slicing and serving with a baby spinach salad.

Hot Okra

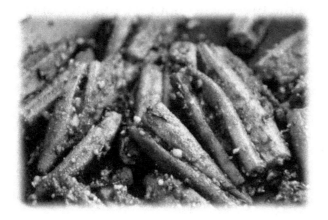

Preparation time: 10 minutes

Cooking time: 20 minutes

Servings: 4

Nutritional Values (Per Serving):

- Calories 182
- Fat 4
- Fiber 2

- Carbs 6
- Protein 6

Ingredients:

- 1 pound okra, halved
- 2 tablespoons avocado oil
- 4 scallions, chopped
- 2 garlic cloves, minced
- 1 tablespoon chili powder
- 1 teaspoon hot paprika
- 1 tablespoon balsamic vinegar
- A pinch of salt and black pepper

Directions:

1. Heat up a pan with the oil over medium heat, add the scallions and the garlic and sauté for 5 minutes.
2. Add the okra and the other ingredients, toss, cook over medium heat for 15 minutes, divide between plates and serve as a side dish.

Hassel-back Potatoes

Preparation time: 10 minutes

Cooking time: 20 minutes

Servings: 4

Nutritional Values (per Serving):

- Calories 355
- Fat 23.4 g
- Carbohydrates 34.5 g
- Sugar 2.5 g
- Protein 4 g
- Cholesterol 61 mg

Ingredients:

- 4 potatoes, wash and dry
- ½ cup butter, melted
- Pepper
- Salt

Directions:

1. Preheat the air fryer to 325 F.
2. Place potato in Hassel back slicer and slice potato using a sharp knife.
3. Brush potatoes with butter and season with pepper and salt.
4. Place potatoes into the air fryer basket and cook for 20 minutes.
5. Serve and enjoy.

Zucchini Carrot Tots

Preparation time: 10 minutes

Cooking time: 10 minutes

Servings: 2

Nutritional Values (per Serving):

- Calories 150
- Fat 5.5 g
- Carbohydrates 16.6 g
- Sugar 4.2 g
- Protein 9.6 g
- Cholesterol 90 mg

Ingredients:

- 1 egg
- 1 carrot, grated & squeeze out the liquid
- 1/4 cup breadcrumbs
- 1 zucchini, grated & squeeze out the liquid

- 1/4 cup parmesan cheese, grated
- ¼ tsp garlic powder
- Pepper
- Salt

Directions:

1. Preheat the air fryer to 400 F.
2. Spray air fryer basket with cooking spray.
3. Add all ingredients into the bowl and mix until well combined.
4. Make tots from mixture and place into the air fryer basket and cook for 10 minutes.
5. Serve and enjoy.

Crispy Green Beans

Preparation time: 10 minutes

Cooking time: 8 minutes

Servings: 2

Nutritional Values (per Serving):

- Calories 245
- Fat 7.1 g
- Carbohydrates 35.5 g
- Sugar 2.7 g
- Protein 10 g
- Cholesterol 89 mg

Ingredients:

- 1 egg, lightly beaten
- 1/2 lb green beans, stem removed
- ¼ tsp Italian seasoning
- 1 cup breadcrumbs

- Pepper
- Salt

Directions:

1. Preheat the air fryer to 400 F.
2. Spray air fryer basket with cooking spray.
3. Add egg to a shallow dish.
4. In a separate dish, mix breadcrumbs, Italian seasoning, pepper, and salt.
5. Dip green beans in egg then coat with breadcrumbs and place into the air fryer basket and cook for 8 minutes.
6. Serve and enjoy.

Flavors Baby Potatoes

Preparation time: 10 minutes

Cooking time: 20 minutes

Servings: 2

Nutritional Values (per Serving):

- Calories 135
- Fat 3.8 g
- Carbohydrates 22 g
- Sugar 0.2 g
- Protein 4.6 g
- Cholesterol 0 mg

Ingredients:

- 12 oz baby potatoes
- 1/4 tsp ground cumin
- 1/4 tsp paprika
- 1/4 tsp chili powder

- 1/2 tbsp butter, melted
- 1/4 tsp pepper
- 1/2 tsp kosher salt

Directions:

1. Preheat the air fryer to 370 F.
2. Add all ingredients into the bowl and toss well.
3. Transfer potatoes into the air fryer basket and cook for 20 minutes. Stir halfway through.
4. Serve and enjoy.

Simple Carrot Fries

Preparation time: 10 minutes

Cooking time: 15 minutes

Servings: 2

Nutritional Values (per Serving):

- Calories 80
- Fat 3.6 g
- Carbohydrates 11.7 g
- Sugar 5.7 g
- Protein 1.1 g
- Cholesterol 0 mg

Ingredients:

- 1/2 lb carrots, peeled and cut into fries shape
- 1/4 tsp ground cumin
- 1/2 tbsp olive oil
- 1/4 tsp paprika

- 1/2 tsp kosher salt

Directions:

1. Preheat the air fryer to 400 F.
2. In a large bowl, add all ingredients and toss until well coated.
3. Transfer carrot fries into the air fryer basket and cook for 15 minutes. Stir halfway through.
4. Serve and enjoy.

Avocado and Cucumber Salad

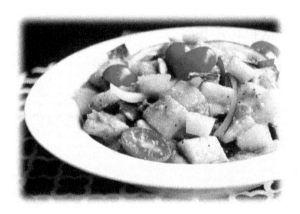

Preparation time: 10 minutes

Cooking time: 0 minutes

Servings: 4

Nutritional Values (Per Serving):

- Calories – 140
- Fat – 4
- Fiber – 2

- Carbs – 4
- Protein - 5

Ingredients:

- 1 onion, peeled and sliced
- 1 cucumber, sliced
- 2 avocados, pitted, peeled, and chopped
- 1 pound cherry tomatoes, halved
- 2 tablespoons olive oil
- ¼ cup fresh cilantro, chopped
- 2 tablespoons lemon juice
- Salt and ground black pepper, to taste

Directions:

1. In a large salad bowl, mix the tomatoes with the cucumber, onion, and avocado, and stir.
2. Add the oil, salt, pepper, and lemon juice, and toss to coat well.
3. Serve cold with cilantro on top.

Arugula Salad

Preparation time: 10 minutes

Cooking time: 0 minutes

Servings: 4

Nutritional Values (Per Serving):

- Calories – 200
- Fat – 2
- Fiber – 1
- Carbs – 5
- Protein - 7

Ingredients:

- 1 white onion, peeled and chopped
- 1 tablespoon vinegar
- 1 cup hot water
- 1 bunch baby arugula
- ¼ cup walnuts, chopped

- 2 tablespoons fresh cilantro, chopped
- 2 garlic cloves, peeled and minced
- 2 tablespoons olive oil
- Salt and ground black pepper, to taste
- 1 tablespoon lemon juice

Directions:

1. In a bowl, mix the water with vinegar, add the onion, set aside for 5 minutes, and drain well.
2. In a salad bowl, mix the arugula with the walnuts and onion, and stir.
3. Add the garlic, salt, pepper, lemon juice, cilantro, and oil, toss well, and serve.

Arugula Soup

Preparation time: 10 minutes

Cooking time: 13 minutes

Servings: 6

Nutritional Values (Per Serving):

- Calories – 200
- Fat – 4
- Fiber – 2
- Carbs – 6
- Protein - 10

Ingredients:

- 1 onion, peeled and chopped
- 1 tablespoon olive oil
- 2 garlic cloves, peeled and minced
- ½ cup coconut milk
- 10 ounces baby arugula

- 2 tablespoons fresh mint, chopped
- 2 tablespoons fresh tarragon, chopped
- 2 tablespoons fresh parsley, chopped
- 2 tablespoons fresh chives, chopped
- 4 tablespoons coconut milk yogurt
- 6 cups chicken stock
- Salt and ground black pepper, to taste

Directions:

1. Heat up a pot with the oil over medium-high heat, add the onion and garlic, stir, and cook for 5 minutes.
2. Add the stock, and milk, stir, and bring to a simmer.
3. Add the arugula, tarragon, parsley, and mint, stir, and cook for 6 minutes.
4. Add the coconut yogurt, salt, pepper, and chives, stir, cook for 2 minutes, divide into soup bowls, and serve.

Arugula and Broccoli Soup

Preparation time: 10 minutes

Cooking time: 20 minutes

Servings: 4

Nutritional Values (Per Serving):

- Calories – 150
- Fat – 3
- Fiber – 1
- Carbs – 3
- Protein - 7

Ingredients:

- 1 onion, peeled and chopped
- 1 tablespoon olive oil
- 1 garlic clove, peeled and minced
- 1 broccoli head, separated into florets
- Salt and ground black pepper, to taste 2

- ½ cups vegetable stock
- 1 teaspoon cumin
- Juice of ½ lemon
- 1 cup arugula leaves

Directions:

1. Heat up a pot with the oil over medium-high heat, add the onions, stir, and cook for 4 minutes.
2. Add the garlic, stir, and cook for 1 minute.
3. Add the broccoli, cumin, salt, and pepper, stir, and cook for 4 minutes.
4. Add the stock, stir, and cook for 8 minutes.
5. Blend the soup using an immersion blender, add half of the arugula, and blend again.
6. Add the rest of the arugula, stir, and heat up the soup again.
7. Add the lemon juice, stir, ladle into soup bowls, and serve.

Zucchini Cream

Preparation time: 10 minutes

Cooking time: 25 minutes

Servings: 8

Nutritional Values (Per Serving):

- Calories – 160
- Fat – 4
- Fiber – 2
- Carbs – 4
- Protein - 8

Ingredients:

- 6 zucchini, cut in half and sliced
- Salt and ground black pepper, to taste
- 1 tablespoon butter
- 28 ounces vegetable stock
- 1 teaspoon dried oregano

- ½ cup onion, chopped
- 3 garlic cloves, peeled and minced
- 2 ounces Parmesan cheese, grated
- ¾ cup heavy cream

Directions:

1. Heat up a pot with the butter over medium-high heat, add the onion, stir, and cook for 4 minutes.
2. Add the garlic, stir, and cook for 2 minutes.
3. Add the zucchini, stir, and cook for 3 minutes.
4. Add the stock, stir, bring to a boil, and simmer over medium heat for 15 minutes.
5. Add the oregano, salt, and pepper, stir, take off the heat, and blend using an immersion blender.
6. Heat the soup again, add the heavy cream, stir, and bring to a simmer.
7. Add the Parmesan cheese, stir, take off the heat, ladle into bowls, and serve.

Swiss Chard Salad

Preparation time: 10 minutes

Cooking time: 20 minutes

Servings: 4

Nutritional Values (Per Serving):

- Calories – 120
- Fat – 2
- Fiber – 1
- Carbs – 4
- Protein - 8

Ingredients:

- 1 bunch Swiss chard, cut into strips
- 2 tablespoons avocado oil
- 1 onion, peeled and chopped
- A pinch of red pepper flakes
- ¼ cup pine nuts, toasted

- ¼ cup raisins
- 1 tablespoon balsamic vinegar
- Salt and ground black pepper, to taste

Directions:

1. Heat up a pan with the oil over medium heat, add the chard and onions, stir, and cook for 5 minutes.
2. Add the salt, pepper, and pepper flakes, stir, and cook for 3 minutes.
3. Put the raisins in a bowl, add the water to cover them, heat them up in a microwave for 1 minute, set aside for 5 minutes, and drain them well.
4. Add the raisins, and pine nuts to the pan with the vinegar, stir, cook for 3 minutes, divide on plates, and serve.

Three Bean Soup

Preparation time: 5 Minutes

Cooking time: 52 Minutes

Servings: 4 To 6

Ingredients:

- 2 tablespoons olive oil
- 1 medium onion, chopped
- 1 medium carrot, chopped
- 1 cup chopped celery
- 2 garlic cloves, minced
- 1 (14.5-ounce) can diced tomatoes, drained
- 1½ cups cooked or 1 (15.5-ounce) can dark red kidney beans, drained and rinsed
- 1½ cups cooked or 1 (15.5-ounce) can black beans, drained and rinsed

- 1½ cups cooked or 1 (15.5-ounce) can navy or other white beans, drained and rinsed
- 4 cups vegetable broth (homemade, store-bought or water)
- 1 tablespoon soy sauce
- 1 teaspoon dried thyme
- 1 bay leaf
- Salt and freshly ground black pepper
- 2 tablespoons chopped fresh parsley

Directions:

1. In a large soup pot, heat the oil over medium heat. Add the onion, carrot, celery, and garlic. Cover and cook until softened, about 7 minutes. Uncover, and stir in the tomatoes, all the beans, and the broth. Add the soy sauce, thyme, and bay leaf and season with salt and pepper to taste. Bring to a boil, then reduce heat to low and simmer until the vegetables are tender, about 45 minutes.
2. Remove the bay leaf and discard before serving. Add the parsley and serve.

Creamy Potato-Cauliflower Soup

Preparation time: 10 Minutes

Cooking time: 25 Minutes

Servings: 6

Nutrition per Serving (2 cups):

- Calories: 80
- Protein: 2g
- Total fat: 1g
- Saturated fat: 0g
- Carbohydrates: 17g
- Fiber: 3g

Ingredients:

- 1 teaspoon olive oil 1 onion, chopped
- 3 cups chopped cauliflower

- 2 potatoes, scrubbed or peeled and chopped
- 6 cups water or Economical Vegetable Broth
- 2 tablespoons dried herbs
- Salt
- Freshly ground black pepper
- 1 or 2 scallions, white and light green parts only, sliced

Directions:

1. Heat the olive oil in a large soup pot over medium-high heat.

2. Add the onion and cauliflower, and sauté for about 5 minutes, until the vegetables are slightly softened. Add the potatoes, water, and dried herbs, and season to taste with salt and pepper. Bring the soup to a boil, reduce the heat to low, and cover the pot. Simmer for 15 to 20 minutes, until the potatoes are soft.

3. Using a hand blender, purée the soup until smooth. (Alternatively, let it cool slightly, then transfer to a countertop blender.) Stir in the scallions and serve. Leftovers will keep in an airtight container for up to 1 week in the refrigerator or up to 1 month in the freezer.

Spicy Pinto Bean Soup

Preparation time: 5 Minutes

Cooking time: 25 Minutes

Servings: 4

Ingredients:

- 1medium onion, chopped
- 1/4 cup chopped celery
- 2garlic cloves, minced
- 1/2 teaspoon ground cumin
- 1/2 teaspoon dried oregano
- 4 cups vegetable broth, (homemade, store-bought or water)
- Salt and freshly ground black pepper
- 2 tablespoons chopped fresh cilantro, for garnish
- 41/2 cups cooked or 3 (15.5-ounce) cans pinto beans, drained and rinsed
- 1 (14.5-ounce) can crushed tomatoes

- 1 teaspoon chipotle chile in adobo
- 2 tablespoons olive oil

Directions:

1. In a food processor, puree 1½ cups of the pinto beans with the tomatoes and chipotle. Set aside.
2. In a large soup pot, heat the oil over medium heat. Add the onion, celery, and garlic. Cover and cook until soft, stirring occasionally, about 10 minutes. Stir in the cumin, oregano, broth, pureed bean mixture, and the remaining 3 cups beans. Season with salt and pepper to taste.
3. Bring to a boil and reduce heat to low and simmer, uncovered, stirring occasionally, until the flavors are incorporated and the soup is hot, about 15 minutes. Ladle into bowls, garnish with cilantro, and serve.

KETO PASTA

Tofu Avocado Keto Noodles

Preparation time: 15 minutes

Serving: 4

Nutritional Values (Per Serving):

- Calories:209
- Total Fat:15.2g
- Saturated Fat:7.3g
- Total Carbs:8g
- Dietary Fiber:1g
- Sugar:2g
- Protein:13g
- Sodium:468mg

Ingredients:

- 2 tbsp butter

- 1 lb tofu
- Salt and black pepper to taste
- 8 large red and yellow bell peppers, Blade A, noodles trimmed 1 tsp garlic powder
- 2 medium avocados, pitted, peeled and mashed
- 2 tbsp chopped pecans for topping

Directions:

1. Melt the butter in a large skillet and cook the tofu until brown, 5 minutes. Season with salt and black pepper.
2. Stir in the bell peppers, garlic powder and cook until the peppers are slightly tender, 2 minutes.
3. Mix in the mashed avocados, adjust the taste with salt and black pepper and cook for 1 minute.
4. Dish the food onto serving plates, garnish with the pecans and serve warm.

Pear and Arugula Salad

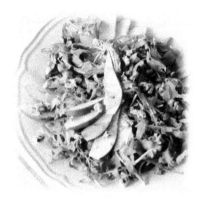

Preparation time: 10 Minutes

Cooking time: 8 Minutes

Servings: 4

Ingredients:

- ¼ cup chopped pecans
- 10 ounces arugula
- 2 pears, thinly sliced
- 1 tablespoon finely minced shallot

- 2 tablespoons champagne vinegar
- 2 tablespoons olive oil
- ¼ teaspoon sea salt
- ¼ teaspoon freshly ground black pepper
- ¼ teaspoon dijon mustard

Directions:

1. Preheat the oven to 350°F.
2. Spread the pecans in a single layer on a baking sheet. Toast in the preheated oven until fragrant, about 6 minutes. Remove from the oven and let cool. In a large bowl, toss the pecans, arugula, and pears. In a small bowl, whisk together the shallot, vinegar, olive oil, salt, pepper, and mustard. Toss with the salad and serve immediately.

Quinoa Salad with Black Beans and Tomatoes

Preparation time: 5 Minutes

Cooking time: 20 Minutes

Servings: 4

Ingredients:

- 3 cups water
- 1½ cups quinoa, well rinsed
- Salt
- 1½ cups cooked or 1 (15.5-ounce) can black beans, drained and rinsed
- 4 ripe plum tomatoes, cut into ¼-inch dice
- ⅓ cup minced red onion
- ¼ cup chopped fresh parsley
- ¼ cup olive oil
- 2 tablespoons sherry vinegar
- ¼ teaspoon freshly ground black pepper

Directions:

1. In a large saucepan, bring the water to boil over high heat. Add the quinoa, salt the water, and return to a boil. Reduce heat to low, cover, and simmer until the water is absorbed, about 20 minutes.

2. Transfer the cooked quinoa to a large bowl. Add the black beans, tomatoes, onion, and parsley.

3. In a small bowl, combine the olive oil, vinegar, salt to taste, and pepper. Pour the dressing over the salad and toss well to combine. Cover and set aside for 20 minutes before serving.

Mediterranean Quinoa Salad

Preparation time: 5 Minutes

Cooking time: 20 Minutes

Servings: 4

Ingredients:

- 2 cups water
- 1 cup quinoa, well rinsed
- Salt
- 1½ cups cooked or 1 (15.5-ounce) can chickpeas, drained and rinsed
- 1 cup ripe grape or cherry tomatoes, halved
- 2 green onions, minced
- ½ medium English cucumber, peeled and chopped
- ¼ cup pitted brine-cured black olives
- 2 tablespoons toasted pine nuts
- ¼ cup small fresh basil leaves
- 1 medium shallot, chopped
- 1 garlic clove, chopped

- 1 teaspoon Dijon mustard
- 2 tablespoons white wine vinegar
- ¼ cup olive oil
- Freshly ground black pepper

Directions:

1. In a large saucepan, bring the water to boil over high heat. Add the quinoa, salt the water, and return to a boil. Reduce heat to low, cover, and simmer until water is absorbed, about 20 minutes.
2. Transfer the cooked quinoa to a large bowl. Add the chickpeas, tomatoes, green onions, cucumber, olives, pine nuts, and basil. Set aside.
3. In a blender or food processor, combine the shallot, garlic, mustard, vinegar, oil, and salt and pepper to taste. Process until well blended. Pour the dressing over the salad, toss gently to combine, and serve.

Apple, Pecan, and Arugula Salad

Preparation time: 10 Minutes

Cooking time: 0 Minutes

Servings: 4

Ingredients:

- Juice of 1 lemon
- 2 tablespoons olive oil
- 1 tablespoon maple syrup
- 2 pinches sea salt
- 1 (5-ounce) package arugula
- 1 cup frozen (and thawed) or fresh corn kernels
- ½ red onion, thinly sliced
- 2 apples (preferably Gala or Fuji), cored and sliced
- ½ cup chopped pecans
- ¼ cup dried cranberries

Directions:

1. In a small bowl, whisk together the lemon juice, oil, maple syrup, and salt. In a large bowl, combine the arugula, corn, red onion, and apples. Add the lemon-juice mixture and toss to combine.

2. Divide evenly among 4 plates and top with the pecans and cranberries.

Healthy Cashew Nuts

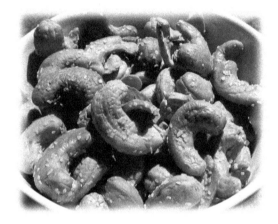

Preparation time: 10 minutes

Cooking time: 6 minutes

Servings: 2

Nutritional Values (per Serving):

- Calories 414
- Fat 34 g
- Carbohydrates 22.8 g

- Sugar 3.5 g
- Protein 10.6 g
- Cholesterol 5 mg

Ingredients:

- 1 cup cashews
- 1 tsp ghee, melted
- ½ tsp chili powder
- Salt

Directions:

1. In a bowl, toss cashews with chili powder, ghee, and salt until well coated.
2. Add cashews into the air fryer basket and roast at 350 F for 5 minutes.
3. Toss cashews and roast for 1 minute more.

Nutritious Fox Nuts

Preparation time: 10 minutes

Cooking time: 10 minutes

Servings: 2

Nutritional Values (per Serving):

- Calories 137
- Fat 6.9 g
- Carbohydrates 15.8 g
- Sugar 0 g
- Protein 3.8 g
- Cholesterol 16 mg

Ingredients:

- 1 1/2 cups fox nuts
- 1/8 tsp turmeric powder
- 1/4 tsp ground black pepper

- 1 tbsp ghee, melted
- Salt

Directions:

1. Preheat the air fryer to 350 F.
2. Add fox nuts, turmeric powder, pepper, salt, and melted ghee in a bowl and mix well.
3. Add fox nuts into the air fryer basket and cook for 10 minutes.
4. Serve and enjoy.

Potato Patties

Preparation time: 10 minutes

Cooking time: 12 minutes

Servings: 5

Nutritional Values (per Serving):

- Calories 80
- Fat 0.4 g
- Carbohydrates 17.5 g
- Sugar 1.9 g
- Protein 1.9 g
- Cholesterol 0 mg

Ingredients:

- 2 potatoes, cooked, peel & mashed
- 2 tbsp cornflour
- ½ tsp ground cumin
- ¼ tsp turmeric

- 1 tbsp ginger garlic paste
- 1 small onion, chopped
- 1 tsp green chili paste
- Salt

Directions:

1. Add all ingredients into the bowl and mix until well combined.
2. Preheat the air fryer to 350 F.
3. Spray air fryer basket with cooking spray.
4. Make equal shapes of patties from the mixture and place them into the air fryer basket and cook for 12 minutes. Turn patties halfway through.
5. Serve and enjoy.

Broccoli Bites

Preparation time: 10 minutes

Cooking time: 15 minutes

Servings: 4

Nutritional Values (per Serving):

- Calories 137
- Fat 2.1 g
- Carbohydrates 12.5 g
- Sugar 4.8 g
- Protein 17.1 g
- Cholesterol 5 mg

Ingredients:

- 2 cups cottage cheese, grated
- 1 cup broccoli, minced
- ½ tsp turmeric
- ¼ cup chickpea flour

- ½ tsp chili powder
- 1 tbsp ginger garlic paste
- Salt

Directions:

1. Add grated cottage cheese, broccoli, and remaining ingredients into the bowl and mix until well combined.
2. Preheat the air fryer to 400 F.
3. Spray air fryer basket with cooking spray.
4. Make small balls from cottage cheese mixture and place them into the air fryer basket and cook for 15 minutes. Turn balls halfway through.
5. Serve and enjoy.

Corn on the Cob

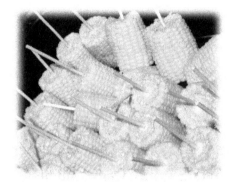

Preparation time: 10 minutes

Cooking time: 20 minutes

Servings: 4

Nutritional Values (per Serving):

- Calories 157
- Fat 4.7 g
- Carbohydrates 29 g
- Sugar 5 g
- Protein 5 g
- Cholesterol 8 mg

Ingredients:

- 4 ears of corn, husked
- 1 tbsp butter, melted
- ½ lemon juice
- Salt

Directions:

1. Brush corn with melted butter and season with salt.
2. Preheat the air fryer to 400 F.
3. Place corn into the air fryer basket and cook for 15-20 minutes.
4. Drizzle lemon juice over corn and serve.

Crispy Okra

Preparation time: 10 minutes

Cooking time: 12 minutes

Servings: 4

Nutritional Values (per Serving):

- Calories 143
- Fat 0.7 g
- Carbohydrates 29.4 g
- Sugar 1.1 g
- Protein 4 g
- Cholesterol 0 mg

Ingredients:

- 10 oz okra, wash & pat dry
- ¼ cup semolina
- ½ cup rice flour
- 1 cup water

- ¾ tsp chili powder
- ½ tsp turmeric
- ½ tsp ground cumin
- Salt

Directions:

1. Slice okra lengthwise in quarters.
2. In a bowl, add rice flour, ground cumin, semolina, turmeric, chili powder, and salt and mix well.
3. Slowly pour water into the rice flour mixture and mix until a thick batter is formed.
4. Add okra into the batter and mix until well coated and set aside for 10 minutes.
5. Spray air fryer basket with cooking spray.
6. Preheat the air fryer to 330 F.
7. Place okra into the air fryer basket and cook for 10 minutes.
8. Remove air fryer basket and shake the okra and cook at 350 F for 2 minutes more.
9. Serve and enjoy.

Walnuts Cream

Preparation time: 10 minutes

Cooking time: 0 minutes

Servings: 4

Nutritional Values (Per Serving):

- Calories 283
- Fat 11.8
- Fiber 0.3
- Carbs 4.7
- Protein 7.1

Ingredients:

- Juice of 1 lime
- ½ cup stevia
- 3 cups coconut milk

- ½ cup coconut cream
- ½ cup walnuts, chopped
- 2 teaspoons cardamom, ground
- 1 teaspoon vanilla extract

Directions:

In a blender, combine the cream with the coconut milk, the walnuts and the other ingredients, pulse well, divide into cups and serve cold.

Avocado Cupcakes

Preparation time: 10 minutes

Cooking time: 20 minutes

Servings: 4

Nutritional Values (Per Serving):

- Calories 142
- Fat 5.8
- Fiber 4.2
- Carbs 5.7
- Protein 1.6

Ingredients:

- 3 tablespoons avocado oil
- 3 tablespoons flaxseed mixed with 4 tablespoons water
- ½ cup coconut milk
- 2 teaspoons cinnamon powder
- 2 avocados, peeled, pitted and chopped

- ¾ cup coconut flour
- ½ teaspoon baking powder
- Cooking spray

Directions:

1. In a bowl, combine the avocado oil with the flaxseed mix, the milk and the other ingredients except the cooking spray, whisk well, pour in a cupcake pan greased with the cooking spray, introduce in the oven at 360 degrees F and bake for 25 minutes.
2. Cool the cupcakes down and serve.

Rhubarb and Berries Cream

Preparation time: 10 minutes

Cooking time: 0 minutes

Servings: 4

Nutritional Values (Per Serving):

- Calories 200
- Fat 5.2
- Fiber 3.4
- Carbs 7.6
- Protein 2.5

Ingredients:

- 2 cups rhubarb, chopped
- 1 cup stevia
- 1 cup blackberries
- 1 teaspoon vanilla extract
- 1 tablespoon avocado oil

- 1/3 cup coconut cream

Directions:

1. In a blender, combine the rhubarb with the stevia, the berries and the rest of the ingredients, pulse well, divide into cups and serve cold.

Rice Pudding

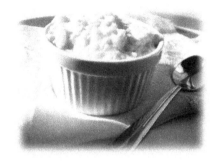

Preparation time: 10 minutes

Cooking time: 20 minutes

Servings: 4

Nutritional Values (Per Serving):

- Calories 234
- Fat 9.5
- Fiber 3.4
- Carbs 12.4
- Protein 6.5

Ingredients:

- 1 cup cauliflower rice 2 cups coconut milk
- 1 cup coconut cream
- 1 teaspoon vanilla extract
- ½ cup stevia
- 1 tablespoon cinnamon powder
- ½ cup avocado, peeled, pitted and cubed

Directions:

1. In a pot, mix the cauliflower rice with the milk, the cream and the other ingredients, stir, bring to a simmer and cook for 20 minutes.
2. Divide into bowls and serve.

Strawberry Sorbet

Preparation time: 3 hours

Cooking time: 10 minutes

Servings: 4

Nutritional Values (Per Serving):

- Calories 182
- Fat 5.4
- Fiber 3.4
- Carbs 12
- Protein 5.4

Ingredients:

- 2 cups coconut water
- 1 cup stevia
- 1 teaspoon vanilla extract
- 1 teaspoon lime zest, grated
- 1 pound strawberries, halved

Directions:

1. Heat up a pan with the coconut water over medium heat, add berries, stevia and the other ingredients, whisk, simmer for 10 minutes, transfer to a blender, pulse, divide into bowls and keep in the freezer for 3 hours before serving.

Cranberries and Avocado Pie

Preparation time: 10 minutes

Cooking time: 40 minutes

Servings: 4

Nutritional Values (Per Serving):

- Calories 172
- Fat 3.4
- Fiber 4.3
- Carbs 11.5
- Protein 4.5

Ingredients:

- 1 cup cranberries
- 1 cup avocado, peeled, pitted and mashed
- 1 cup coconut cream
- 1 cup stevia Cooking spray
- 1/3 cup almond flour

- 1 cup coconut, unsweetened and shredded
- ¼ cup avocado oil

Directions:

1. In a bowl, mix the cranberries with the avocado, the cream and the other ingredients except the cooking spray and whisk well.
2. Grease a cake pan with the cooking spray, pour the pie mix inside and bake at 350 degrees F for 40 minutes.
3. Cool the pie down, slice and serve.

Lime Cream

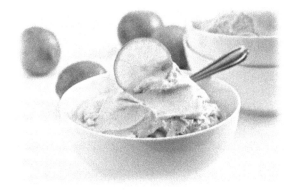

Preparation time: 1 hour

Cooking time: 0 minutes

Servings: 6

Nutritional Values (Per Serving):

- Calories 200
- Fat 8.5
- Fiber 4.5
- Carbs 8.6
- Protein 4.5

Ingredients:

- 2 tablespoons flaxseed mixed with 3 tablespoons water
- 1 cup stevia
- 5 tablespoons avocado oil
- 1 cup coconut cream
- Juice of 1 lime
- Zest of 1 lime, grated

Directions:

1. In a blender, combine the flaxseed mix with the stevia, the oil and the other ingredients, pulse well, divide into cups and keep in the fridge for 1 hour before serving.

Cherries Stew

Preparation time: 10 minutes

Cooking time: 10 minutes

Servings: 4

Nutritional Values (Per Serving):

- Calories 192
- Fat 5.4
- Fiber 3.4
- Carbs 9.4
- Protein 4.5

Ingredients:

- 2 cups cherries, pitted
- 3 tablespoons stevia
- 2 cups water
- 1 tablespoon mint, chopped
- 1 teaspoon vanilla extract

Directions:

1. In a pan, combine the cherries with the stevia, water and the other ingredients, stir, bring to a simmer and cook over medium-low heat for 10 minutes.
2. Divide into cups and serve cold.

Chocolate Fudge

Preparation time: 10 minutes

Cooking time: 0 minute

Servings: 12

Nutritions:

- Calories 157
- Fat 14.1g
- Carbohydrates 6.1g
- Sugar 1g
- Protein 2.3g
- Cholesterol 0mg

Ingredients:

- 4 oz unsweetened dark chocolate
- 3/4 cup coconut butter

- 15 drops liquid stevia
- 1 tsp vanilla extract

Directions:

1. Melt coconut butter and dark chocolate.
2. Add ingredients to the large bowl and combine well.
3. Pour mixture into a silicone loaf pan and place in refrigerator until set.
4. Cut into pieces and serve.

Coconut Peanut Butter Fudge

Preparation time: 10 minutes

Cooking time: 0 minute

Servings: 12

Nutritions:

- Calories 125
- Fat 11.3g
- Carbohydrates 3.5g
- Sugar 1.7g
- Protein 4.3g
- Cholesterol 0mg

Ingredients:

- 12 oz smooth peanut butter
- 3 tbsp coconut oil
- 4 tbsp coconut cream
- 15 drops liquid stevia

- Pinch of salt

Directions:

1. Line baking tray with parchment paper.
2. Melt coconut oil in a saucepan over low heat.
3. Add peanut butter, coconut cream, stevia, and salt in a saucepan. Stir well.
4. Pour fudge mixture into the prepared baking tray and place in refrigerator for 1 hour.
5. Cut into pieces and serve.

Raspberry Chia Pudding

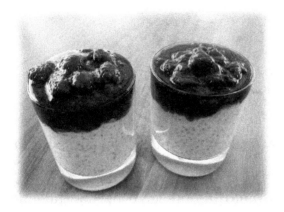

Preparation time: 3 hours & 10 minutes

Cooking time: 0 minute

Servings: 2

Nutritions:

- Calories 361
- Fat 33.4g
- Carbohydrates 13.3g
- Sugar 5.4g
- Protein 6.2g
- Cholesterol 0mg

Ingredients:

- 4 tbsp chia seeds
- 1 cup coconut milk
- 1/2 cup raspberries

Directions:

1. Add raspberry and coconut milk in a blender and blend until smooth.
2. Pour mixture into the Mason jar.
3. Add chia seeds in a jar and stir well.
4. Close jar tightly with lid and shake well.
5. Place in refrigerator for 3 hours.
6. Serve chilled and enjoy.

Quick Choco Brownie

Preparation time: 10 minutes

Cooking time: 0 minute

Servings: 1

Nutritions:

- Calories 207
- Fat 15.8g
- Carbohydrates 9.5g
- Sugar 3.1g
- Protein 12.4g
- Cholesterol 20mg

Ingredients:

- 1/4 cup almond milk
- 1 tbsp cocoa powder
- 1 scoop chocolate protein powder
- 1/2 tsp baking powder

Directions:

1. In a microwave-safe mug blend together baking powder, protein powder, and cocoa.
2. Add almond milk in a mug and stir well.
3. Place mug in microwave and microwave for 30 seconds.
4. Serve and enjoy.

Choco Chia Pudding

Preparation time: 10 minutes

Cooking time: 0 minute

Servings: 6

Nutritions:

- Calories 259
- Fat 25.4g
- Carbohydrates 10.2g
- Sugar 3.5g
- Protein 3.8g
- Cholesterol 0mg

Ingredients:

- 2 1/2 cups coconut milk
- 2 scoops stevia extract powder
- 6 tbsp cocoa powder
- 1/2 cup chia seeds

- 1/2 tsp vanilla extract
- 1/8 cup xylitol
- 1/8 tsp salt

Directions:

1. Add all ingredients into the blender and blend until smooth.
2. Pour mixture into the glass container and place in refrigerator.
3. Serve chilled and enjoy.

Smooth Chocolate Mousse

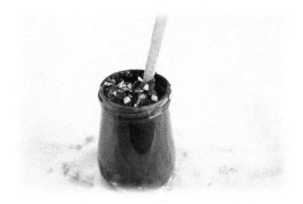

Preparation time: 10 minutes

Cooking time: 0 minute

Servings: 2

Nutritions:

- Calories 296
- Fat 29.7g
- Carbohydrates 11.5g
- Sugar 4.2g
- Protein 4.4g
- Cholesterol 0mg

Ingredients:

- 1/2 tsp cinnamon
- 3 tbsp unsweetened cocoa powder
- 1 cup creamed coconut milk
- 10 drops liquid stevia

Directions:

1. Place coconut milk can in the refrigerator for overnight; it should get thick and the solids separate from water.
2. Transfer thick part into the large mixing bowl without water.
3. Add remaining ingredients to the bowl and whip with electric mixer until smooth.
4. Serve and enjoy.

CPSIA information can be obtained
at www.ICGtesting.com
Printed in the USA
LVHW022342080621
689681LV00006B/620

9 781802 772258